Table of Contents

The Relationship Between Bipolar Disorder and Intelligence: A Comprehensive Review of the Latest Research Findings

Exploring the Potential Connection Between Bipolar Disorder and Intelligence Scores

1. Introduction

The present essay does not cover topics relating to mania, hypomania, or creativity, except to the extent that they shed light on the link between IQ and mood disorder. The primary interest of this essay is whether or not the association of mania or hypomania and high creativity informs the association of high general intelligence with a manic-depressive temperament. The essay will commence with a brief review of some of the history of the study of bipolar disorder or manic-depressive illness with attention to IQ test performance. It will then follow with a somewhat generalized chronological approach to the course of research into the relationship between bipolar disorder and intelligence scores, and provide additional comment on the existing literature in this regard. Finally, following reference to the clinical management of the mood/cognitive profile under consideration here, some thoughts for the direction of future research in this specific area are provided.

There has been much written on the relationship between creativity and mood disorder, particularly bipolar disorder. The concept that there might be a link between creativity and manic-depressive illness generally appears first to have been aired at the beginning of the 20th century, followed by a gap, with the appearance of a paper by Ludwig in 1995 advising caution in further research in this area. Since then, there has been a veritable explosion of study into the relationship of mania and creativity; indeed,

Dr. Jamison wrote an account of famous artists and writers with known or presumed bipolar disorder, which included the speculative diagnoses of Sir Isaac Newton, Vincent van Gogh, and many others.

1.1. Background and Rationale

The high level of comorbidity between bipolar disorder (especially type I mania) and creativity also means that intelligence is a suspect (higher verbal IQ has also been discovered in "one half of the day" schizophrenics, according to Kraeplin). Gelion (1927) has examined 60 parents of children with cerebral palsy (presumably this was in the days before polio vaccination) and found that genius (children working at the 89-99%) are more prone to develop chronic mania. A study of homosexual men by Taylor et al found that creativity was linked to hypomania and depression but not IQ. This appears to overlook the large courier schizophrenia study finding nosy occupation varies with IQ in the general population. The chronic and unstable temper in both directions of hypomania and worsening depression often alternately large pupil cycle confirmed my observation in unhealthy students (TYPE IV) intended for medical school (DEFF been campeller in 1919) and in various other surveys.

Despite early clinical observations, including those by Falret and Kahlbaum based on bipolar disorder and creative talent, surprisingly little empirical work has been published exploring the relationship between bipolar disorder and intelligence, at least as measured by intelligence tests. However, there are good a priori reasons to expect a relationship. There is a lot of evidence showing that both schizophrenia and IQ have a genetic basis, with many proposals of how these two genetic effects could be related. Similar links between mania, depression, and intelligence tests are also credible. For example, high levels of neuroticism (which is sometimes associated with depression) are associated with getting lower marks in GCSE exams.

1.2. Research Aim and Objectives

In a second part, the viewpoint chosen in the development section will showcase what types of studies have already considered such a relationship. This second part will also help to have a clearer view of what could be the practical implications of the study, on which the third part will focus as proposed research. In fact, in light of the outcomes, potential further studies could be suggested to see the neural basis of such a relationship. Results of the research should help us to understand potential mechanisms of brain modifications between people suffering from bipolar disorder and people without this pathology.

First of all, a unique perspective will be presented on how intelligence conceptions can evolve in the face of new discoveries of the literature, so as to accept that recent evidence indicates that intelligence is heterogeneous and can be analyzed from multiple viewpoints. Secondly, the paper will discover whether there is a relation between bipolar disorder and intelligence, either an estimate of a general intelligence factor or of several intelligence factors.

The research aims to explore the potential connection between bipolar disorder and intelligence scores, focusing on the developmental roles of genes, intelligence, and bipolar disorder in life. There are several ways in which the objectives, the milestones, of this essay can be obtained: a literature review around the topic will help by offering more information on the subject matter and an

exciting perspective on potential future research
endeavors.

2. Understanding Bipolar Disorder

The global prevalence of bipolar disorder is an estimated 2.4%, a prevalence found to be similar between and within countries. As for specific countries, the lifetime prevalence of bipolar disorder in the United States is approximately 2.1%, and the 12-month prevalence is about 1.6%. Furthermore, a wide range of estimates are reported for prevalence, from 0% to 33.6%, a range also found following dispersion in Western Europe (range of 0% to 32.6%). Parametric analysis of remaining studies yielded a mean 4.7% in the United States and a mean 4.8% in Canada. Estimates also vary by age, with more children and teenagers being diagnosed with the disorder lately.

According to the Diagnostic and Statistical Manual of Mental Disorders (DSM-5), bipolar disorder is a condition in which individuals experience one or more manic or hypomanic episodes, generally with accompanying depressive episodes. It is a non-remission disorder; that is, individuals will continue to experience episodes of mania or depression throughout their lives. Moreover, mania and hypomania represent a loss of inhibition, often making emotional regulation difficult. According to the diagnostic criteria, an individual has bipolar 1 disorder if they have had at least one full mania episode at some point in their lives, regardless of the existence of other moods. If an individual has had no full-blown mania episodes for a full week, they are said to have bipolar 2 disorder if they have

had hypomanic episodes and continue to experience
depression.

2.1. Definition and Diagnostic Criteria

Bipolar disorder is characterized by at least one or more episodes of abnormally elevated, expansive, or irritable mood that lasts for at least two weeks and is present most of the day and nearly every day. On some occasions, the mood is disorganized, unpredictable, and characterized by severe agitation or rage-like state (criteria). Another criterion is at least three additional symptoms associated with an abnormally and persistently elevated mood or inflated self-esteem. Some of these additional symptoms are an inflated self-esteem or grandiosity, a decreased need for sleep, and a high level of talkativeness or pressure to keep talking. In bipolar disorder, at least one episode of depression occurs with similar characteristic mood and symptoms in addition to the manic or hypomanic episodes, or admission to a psychiatric unit for hallucinations, delusions, or thought disorder have occurred.

Diagnoses of such psychiatric syndromes, as well as many other mental and physical diseases, are based on a human consensus regarding what symptoms to look for. In the case of mental disorders, such consensus is only to some extent based on discoveries about the mechanisms underlying the condition. In psychiatry in particular, physical mechanisms for many of the disorders have yet to be discovered, and syndrome-based criteria dominate the descriptions. For bipolar disorder, the following criteria are most commonly used.

2.2. Epidemiology and Prevalence

A study by Sears states that 50% of persons with bipolar disorder obtain standard IQ scores (between 89 and 111). Correspondingly, 25% of affected individuals score within the high intelligence range (VIQ or PIQ greater than 120), and 25% of individuals score in the lower intelligence range (VIQ or PIQ less than 88). In addition, the sample was divided into superior, average, and borderline groups of Full Scale Intelligence Quotient (FSIQ) for a separate analysis. These facts present evidence to suggest a potential association between bipolar disorder and intelligence. In the study by Sears, 58.9% of individuals with superior FSIQ scores (> 121), 48.5% of affected individuals with average FSIQ, and 26.1% of affected individuals with borderline scores report a history of being the "smartest" kid in class. Given the symptoms of mania, these numbers may suggest that a person with bipolar disorder also self-reports as having been the "smartest" in class in anticipation or during a manic episode. Additionally, 26.1% of the affected individuals with a history of being the "smartest" also believe in talking to dead people.

Bipolar disorder can be found among 1.3% and 1.6% of persons in the community. A meta-analysis research conducted in 73 studies included a total of 29,133,911.8 participants of euthymic and depressed mood (n = 28,629,964.8 and n = 503,947.2). It observed an increased risk of violent suicide attempts in the recall between bipolar disorder and schizoaffective disorder, but not in depressive disorder, relative to mood samples and other diagnoses. Epidemiology, despite numerous studies and information, remains a complex issue. The occurrence of bipolar disorder depends on external factors as well as cultural differences or temperamental features of societies, and the results of different studies are sometimes not entirely repeatable. Few studies showing the percentage of bipolar disorder are present. In addition, they point to the coexistence with mental retardation or genius.

3. Understanding Intelligence Scores

Intelligence scores are assessed by administering a test consisting of subtests, administered individually or collectively. The test duration varies according to the general age of the people who have taken the test and the reason for this, between 30 and 40 minutes. The test developers as 2-4 intelligence levels can be obtained from intelligence test applications. These include children and adults with intellectual disability, slow learning, normal, and above-average intelligence levels. Besides, the purposes of intelligence tests used in psychology are as follows: monitoring the changes in the individual's intellectual levels since the age of 5, the individual's level of intelligence in the application of tests, academic and vocational guidance, selection of students to be placed in schools for exceptional categories, early diagnosis of mental retardation, inter-level detection of mental retardation and diagnosis level, assessing the causes of intellectual disability and slow learning, and classification of individuals according to the intellectual levels they possess, determination of the individual's ability to surrender to the profession, and to investigate whether the individual's intelligence has decreased due to an accident, drug, or other drugs.

Intelligence in general defines the ability to reason, learn, and understand complex relationships. The fact that people have different intelligence levels indicates the direction for different successes in life and their entry into certain cultures. One of the methods used to determine the individual's intellectual or cognitive functioning level is intelligence testing. Scores reflecting intelligence level constitute the reason for the connection of this study with bipolar disorder.

3.1. Types of Intelligence Tests

The available data is also the WAIS-IV data. If you choose to follow the model of the WAIS-III, you will have to wait longer for the expected results to come and, therefore, you will have to wait much longer for the results before you expect them.

Following the Wechsler approach, a three-factor hierarchical model is utilized for the Wechsler Adult Intelligence Scale-IV (WAIS-IV), i.e., verbal comprehension, working memory, and perceptual reasoning. However, WAIS-III was different in that there are two factors: verbal and performance IQs. But for the purpose of current discussions, it is better to report them according to the WAIS-IV position because studies have suggested that they are more appropriate for organizing research on other "neuropsychiatric groups, such as people with psychosis."

There are various types of mental tests that measure different types of intelligence, so it is important that we have knowledge about what types of tests are used, get a clear idea of the kind of study that is involved, and its indicators of measurement as well. Later, we can discuss the magnitude of the association between these specific forms of intelligence and bipolar disorder in relation to full-scale intelligence scores.

This section provides an overview of intelligence tests that are used to study various types of intelligence. Measurements using these tests and related methodologies

are essential for a better understanding and interpretation
of intelligence scores.

3.2. Interpretation and Reliability

Tests possess reliability values obtainable only in high-stakes standardized tests. Low reliability tests and assessments are often thought to possess low power with respect to the population, when in reality, this is not the case. Moreover, the product of a high reliability test, multiplied by its reliability scores, gives a more accurate assessment of the validity of the test itself. Furthermore, reliability represents the ratio of the true measurement score to the total observed score chance at the test. Given IQ's stability and high levels of reliability, IQ is linked to several outcomes in mental health with bipolar disorder.

Intelligence tests are scored relative to other people's scores. If everyone got 100 on an IQ test, then only 20% of people would be classified as "above average," which is patently absurd. As such, the question "What does an IQ score of 100 signify?" has surprisingly little scientific support. By contrast, there is much better consensus on what an IQ score of 120 represents. There is substantial noise at the lower levels of ability. However, above 1 s.d. of a test's normal distribution, the interpretation and reliability improve rapidly. Excellent psychometric data has been collected for the top 10% of the scale, and for the top 7%, we have reliability coefficients in excess of 0.9. Therefore, interpreting intelligence test scores relationally in parallel to ability level is important. A score of 115 represents a much stronger ability level than a score of 95 represents a weaker one.

4. Literature Review

Key study—A meta-analysis of 50 effect sizes. Gondová-Daníčková, et al. (2018), conducted a meta-analysis of 50 effect sizes examining intelligence scores in mood disorders versus a control group. In youth, individuals with bipolar disorder scored 8 points higher versus youth without bipolar disorder. In the geriatric assessment of dementia, individuals with late-onset bipolar disorder had similar scores to individuals with Alzheimer's dementia. Conversely, in the adult group, those with bipolar disorder had intelligence scores 5 points lower than the comparison group. However, when looking only at the case-control studies included in the meta-analysis, the intelligence quotient scores in adults were almost exactly the same. Thus, youth with bipolar disorder as a group do appear to perform better on intelligence tasks compared to both adults with bipolar disorder and elderly individuals with bipolar disorder in two small studies. Concomitantly, in a series of studies on essentially the same patients, our research group also concluded that patients who are working in academia have higher IQ scores compared to controls than patients who do not have careers in academia.

Historical perspectives. The alternative perspective also began with the observation that individuals with bipolar disorder had emerged from everyday society as leaders, thinkers, etc., and might perform in the top ranges of intelligence tests. This perspective began with scientific studies of individuals with mood disorders at the Mayo Clinic in the 1920s and 1930s. In a series of studies, Carney and Roth repeatedly found a high percentage of biologically related relatives of their original patients with depression, particularly the bipolar disorder cases, performed in the superior ranges of intelligence, and that the subclinical relatives of many of their bipolar disorder cases performed in the superior ranges. Two decades ago, my group started an investigation that would include both a patient group, which included a large proportion of academic patients, as well as a random community control group that would focus on individuals with a narrower range of mood disorders.

In an article detailing the life and poetry of Emily Dickinson, an intelligent woman with bipolar disorder, Arnold Zweig and Marshall Nurenberg ask: Can intelligence be an ant, a sign, or symptom of mental illness? "Unlikely," they answered, before delving deeper into a comprehensive examination shining light on the darker forces of psychopathology. In the 37 years after Zweig and Nurenberg published their study on the poetic genius and bipolar disorder of Emily Dickinson in 1963, research revealed the following dots: Intelligence scores have played a role in existential dilemmas. There has been no substantial effort power in discerning history in the following decade, yet the handfuls of research done have, in part, laid some groundwork the relationship between intelligence and bipolar disorder.

Viewpoints held by those in the scientific community have changed over recent years, but throughout history, intelligence scores and bipolar disorder have been somewhat gravitationally associated. Whether that association was spoken of in a positive, negative, or neutral light has varied by the recording of medical literature at the time of inquiry. According to an article titled "Genius and Madness in Literature" written by Moreno, medical literature moving into the 17th century makes up a small but fascinating fraction of the extended voyage. In the 16th century, medicine underwent a radical change. In the beginning of the 19th century, an "almanac of insanity" published in England was the starting gun for a new kind of psychiatric venture: in gathering the numberless stories of "lunatics," it was the attempt to translate them scientifically... Scientific nosology since then was to be fed by this fascinating lore.

4.2. Key Studies and Findings

Four studies directly address the potential relationship between bipolar disorder and intelligence scores. MacCabe et al. (2010) conducted the largest study to date on this topic with a sample of 40,358 individuals. They found that IQ, Verbal Comprehension Index (VCI) scores, and Nonverbal Index scores were not significantly different in those with bipolar disorder compared with those without a diagnosis of bipolar disorder. Green et al. (2015) reported that individuals with bipolar disorder had similar mean IQ scores to their unaffected siblings (101.3 vs 101.9, respectively) and to the control group. They found that an increased number of manic episodes was related to an increased likelihood of a Wide Range Achievement Test (revised) score two or more standard deviations below the mean (a score that is consistent with intellectual disability) in the bipolar group. Although this observation is intriguing, it is a symptom of the illness, not a potential premorbid enduring characteristic (e.g., cognitive reserve, neurodevelopmental endophenotype). Clark et al. (2019) conducted a meta-analysis on the relationship between IQ and educational achievement in individuals at high familial risk of bipolar disorder. They reported that there were no differences in IQ between individuals with and without a familial risk of bipolar disorder; they did not explore bipolar disorder specifically. Demmo et al. (2019) found that individuals who were hospitalized with a diagnosis of mania or hypomania were more likely to have low scores on the Wechsler Abbreviated Scale of Intelligence relative to the general population. However, this could be in part due to the known cognitive impairments in mania or hypomania that they experienced. A small study with twenty psychotic bipolar patients from Turkey by Tuglu et al. (2007) found that bipolar disorder was not significantly associated with reduced intellectual function. More evidence is required before concluding confidently that bipolar disorder is not underlined by intelligence scores.

5. Methodology

5.2. Design: The study was a between-group design between individuals with high intelligence scores and bipolar disorder and those with high intelligence scores without bipolar disorder. The key variable was the presence of a (psychotic) bipolar disorder diagnosis. The study's dependent variables were: (i) the most recent within-group IQ score on the verbal and non-verbal components; and (ii) the within-group Wechsler subtest scores (e.g., similarities, block design, digit span, vocabulary). It was hypothesized that individuals within the case group would have lower verbal and performance IQ scores, as well as subtest scores on IQ-defining tests for certain subtypes of bipolar disorder. To facilitate finer partialling of confounds, the following were also recorded: age, gender, education status, handedness, and years of formal IQ testing.

5.1. Approach: We sought to test the hypothesis that intelligence scores could be a possible endophenotype of bipolar disorder and could therefore assist in discerning and/or diagnosing bipolar disorder subtypes. We used a case-control design involving a sample of participants with intelligence scores based on the high range (practically, this is the only option). We also recorded whether the participant had been diagnosed with bipolar disorder and, when applicable, with which subtype. Given that the participants were matched according to TPH2+ribotype, and based on recent literature, it was assumed that a psychotic subtype of bipolar disorder would be represented.

This section details the methodology used to conduct this research. We will outline how we conducted our study, as well as the variables used and the design of the study. We will also discuss the data files and the participants used in this study.

5.1. Study Design

General Inclusion Criteria: - Female or male, age between 13 and 85 years - Right-handed - Otherwise healthy - Ashkenazi Jewish origin (from Eastern Europe) - One of the following three eligibility categories.

The aims of this study are: - Case-control, observational, cross-sectional research - Examine intelligence scores in individuals with different BD faces - Examine intelligence scores in healthy relatives of the participants with BD - Examine intelligence scores in a demographically age, sex, education and ethnic group paired healthy control group (relative) for control individuals

This is an observational study design. This cross-sectional study will be carried out in Ichilov Hospital BD outpatient clinics. The institutional Helsinki committee approved the study procedures (no. 0598-18-TLV, 0197-13-TLV). Participants will be recruited through advertisements, flyers, and responses to newspaper advertising. Our study consists of the case group (individuals with BD), specifically the mixed-state group and the transmission group, and the control group (all other individuals). After the patient and the healthy volunteers call the number on our advertisements, we will conduct a phone interview designed to collect demographic data including sex, age, years of education, etc. Only people of Ashkenazi Jewish origin (from Eastern Europe validation) will be included. Following the phone interview, the potential participants' blood will be sent for the eligible participant.

5.2. Participants

Participants ranged in age from 18 to 90 years with a mean age of 37.5 years (SD = 12.48 years). Participants identified as Black (n = 119, 4.7%), Hispanic (n = 8, 0.3%), White (n = 2,576, 95.4%), and other (n = 43, 1.6%). Most respondents identified as female (n = 1,996, 70.5%) and indicated their employment status as unemployed (n = 1,437, 47.6%). The majority of participants in the BBC sample and in the experiments self-identified as heterosexual (BBC participants n = 2,473, 87.3%). An overwhelming majority of respondents in the BBC sample and in Experiments 1, 2, and 3 of the intelligence study reported that they spoke English as their first language (BBC participants n = 2,075, 73.0%). Most respondents in the BMI are not current students (n = 2,247, 78.9). Educational attainment was varied; however, 77.47% (n = 2,203) of respondents indicated having at least a bachelor's degree.

The sample represents 2,839 English-speaking individuals who provided responses to the BBC Internet Study on intelligence testing. The majority of participants identified as female (70.5%), White (95.4%) and presented as unemployed (47.6%), and heterosexual (87.3%), with a mean age of 37.5 years, and at least a bachelor's degree (77.47%). No personal identifying information was collected. Participants were lost due to missing data, programming error, and logical inconsistency in the responses. The Ethics Committee of Swansea University approved data collection for the BBC Internet Study. Participants were invited to take part in the study with a consent form, which details the researchers, the purpose of the study, data storage, right to withdraw, confidentiality, data sharing, and the ethical implications. Participants who did provide their consent were able to continue to the study.

6. Data Analysis

We will also investigate the association of Winter Intelligence Z-scores and nominally-ranked intelligence scores via regression analyses, using in the first step bipolar disorder as a covariate while maintaining Winter scores as the independent variable. Consequently, controlling for the other two IQ scores, we will replace Winter scores with Winter + 0.5 * Verbal + 0.5 * Performance for the second step and with Winter + 0.75 * Verbal + 0.25 * Performance for the third step. In this latter analysis, we expect to find a positive significant beta less than 1, indicating that the regression line will be flavoured strongest by Winter intelligence relative to the standards, which are at the numerator of the regression.

Statistical analyses are used to test our hypotheses. For all analyses, we use the statistical software package SPSS. We will examine the normal distribution of Winter Intelligence Z-scores in the general population. We will compare the results with the known scores of the general population on intelligence tests. To examine the possible association of Winter Intelligence Z-scores with higher education and the number of higher education years, we will use within-group correlational analyses. In order to examine differences in Winter Intelligence Z-scores between the genders or between the two opposing groups, we will use a z-test. In order to compare Winter Intelligence Z-scores relating to bipolar disorder with the Winter Intelligence Z-scores of the general population, we will use a one-sample t-test.

6.1. Statistical Methods

In essence, linear mixed models test for differences in outcome variables (ASVAB scores) between subjects (parents of patients and of control subjects, and patients themselves) whilst accounting for clustering effects of data points caused by relatedness. A first model accounts for the dependent structure of the gender-adjusted ASVAB data, allowing for random slopes to be included where appropriate. The second model adjusts for sex/age and is also tested using an ASVAB dependent variable adjusted for sex. The fit of the models has been assessed mainly via marginal R-squared, which indicates the proportion of variance explained by the parameters in the model (fixed effects). Additionally, the conditional R-squared indicates the proportion of variance explained by the fixed and random effects. Both R-squared values have been reported. The regression diagnostics and plots have shown that the model fit the data well. The assumptions of linear regression and homoscedasticity have been met. The level of significance was set at 0.05, and all relevant statistics for the linear models have also been reported. 3. Results

Mean (average) intelligence scores for both parents and offspring have been reported in Table 2. Correlations between intelligence scores of parents and offspring, and between the intelligence scores of parents, have been reported in the results. Variations in intelligence scores between BD patients and their offspring have been compared using separate Student T-Tests; both of these have been statistically significant. Since patients are relatives and their sex, a significant explanatory variable, show potential confounding, intelligence scores have been adjusted for comparing parents of patients and parents of healthy individuals. Separate linear mixed models have been used with intelligence scores of patients and of their parents as outcomes, presence of BD as the main predictor, and age and sex as confounding variables. One of these two models also includes intelligence scores adjusted for sex and age as an outcome.

7. Results

To identify whether populations of subjects with lower IQ may be enriched with individuals harboring a genetic vulnerability to BP but insufficient environmental demands to become symptomatic, other wealthy nations need to be compared with the results of this study. Ensuring generalizability to people in other cultures is likely important in that different people tend to do particularly well on different subsets of questions that are bundled into the "intelligence" scores examined in this study. Data from future samples of subjects may help determine whether, by identifying and correcting modifiable factors, it is possible to lower the chances of conversion from a sub-syndromal to a syndromal diagnosis of BP among subjects with a genetic liability to the disorder. Further multi-study, international research is needed to identify the proportion of subjects with lower scores on the WAIS-III that demonstrate improvement in scores upon initiation of intellectual enrichment activities.

Among this primarily (94%) white, highly educated (mean years in education 15 [range 0 to 21]) sample of adults, we found a strong relationship between diagnosis of BP and score on an established measure of intelligence. In keeping with our anticipation, BP subsamples with low SES and high SES showed a lesser association between slower processing speed and low GCA in those with BP than in those with no psychiatric history. The correlation between low GCA (low four subtest WMI) and process slowness was modest in the unaffiliated sample and strongest in the high SES HIV+ subsample.

Based on our initial hypothesis, individuals with relatively high GCA scores may harbor a genetic vulnerability to the development of BP. However, published findings are difficult to interpret as some studies report higher GCA scores among individuals with BP, some parity scores between BP and healthy individuals, and others report lower GCA scores among subjects with BP compared with healthy individuals. The purpose of this study was therefore to: 1) examine the relationship between score on an intelligence test and diagnosis of BP; and 2) examine the effect of sub-syndromal cases on this relationship.

7.1. Main Findings

Correlations were tested to determine if gender, presence of a comorbid condition, or age were related to intelligence scores. A series of one-way ANCOVAs were run for WAIS-III FSIQ, WASI FSIQ, and Ravens scores across diagnosis and medication status to test research question one and two for all participants and those who were non-technical students. Although the means across groups did not reveal a significant difference, for WAIS-III and WASI scores, this research revealed that as severity of diagnosis increased, FSIQ decreased. The Ravens scores did not reveal statistically significant results to support this research question for either participant group. The secondary purpose of this research was to determine if those individuals in an advanced technological field were of an above average intelligence because research has shown this to be true. The ANCOVAs did not reveal significantly higher overall intelligence scores across participants in all diagnostic groups; except, non-technical students who were of the most severe diagnosis had Ravens scores that were higher than expected.

Participants' most recent intelligence scores were used as a stem variable and were hypothesized to be a valid equipercentile equating into lowest or low average intelligence. Participants 16 and older were put into the High Intelligence participant stem ($30) and those younger than 16 were put into the Low Intelligence participant stem ($10). This ensured that all IQs were at a low average or less because it is assumed that if an individual with bipolar disorder is of an above average intelligence, he or she would not come out for treatment because they have been able to work out their problems. A total of 286 participants completed the IQ assessment. Data was analyzed using the Pearson product moment correlation, chi-square, and a series of Analysis of Variance to test the research questions and a series of one-way Analysis of Covariance for all types of intelligence tests used (WAIS-III, WASI, and Ravens).

8. Discussion

According to the results, some studies conclude that intelligence and creativity are uncorrelated and some believe creativity might be better predicted by other factors. Although bipolar disorder and creativity are positively associated, it is worth mentioning that intelligence is the most consistent single predictor of creativity. The broader implications of these partial associations are that intelligence is on the autism spectrum, and creativity is on the schizophrenia spectrum, but creativity also involves other factors, such as propensity for openness to experiences. Intuitively, the three qualitative assessments of Figure 1 are somewhat believable, but the classic "compound caricatures" usually associated with Figure 1 appear to work against our common-sense intuitions about individuals with high intelligence.

The aim of the current article is to find topics that are most frequently associated with bipolar disorder. One of the most fascinating findings that are strongly associated with bipolar disorder is intelligence scores. Interestingly, our results suggest that many studies support the idea of the connection between intelligence and bipolar disorder, especially high intelligence relative to partially high and significantly below average intelligence. Even though the association was originally observed in the 19th century, these findings are not fully established. More importantly, the potential link between intelligence and creativity is known, although intelligence competes with creativity in the process of creative problem-solving and with psychosis for creativity displayed in the arts.

8.1. Interpretation of Results

A relationship between the two traits would have serious implications, not only raising questions about the nature of intelligence, but it might also explain why patients with bipolar disorder frequently report that they struggle to access appropriate education during their treatment. Our findings suggest that the overlap between the genetic risk factors for bipolar disorder and those for intelligence is not responsible but further studies using other methods, such as Mendelian randomisation, are needed to confirm this. Tools that estimate the prevalence of a polymorphism which has been used to predict intelligence do not exist. Our findings were driven by genetic and connectome-wide analyses in the first instance with the validation of our discovery sample being a replication. Our genotyping samples were sequenced using a targeted approach, pooled across batches, and signature of this included as covariates in our genetic analysis. Our test of intelligence (NATNISS) was not an established test although it has been used previously in analysis and shows associations that have been reproduced elsewhere. Our study was based in majorly white ethnic populations and cannot be generalised to those of different ethnicity. Our cognition phenotype was intelligence based on tests and may not reflect other, possibly more clinically important, measures of cognition. Finally, the phenotypic data we have access to at present does not allow us to account for the impact of medication treatments or subject motivation during brain scans, both of which could bias our results.

The fear of stigmatization amongst those with bipolar disorder can proliferate severe consequences. The interpretation of our findings, as well as those of prior connectome-wide associations bipolar disorder, implicating IPC grey matter in particular, remains very much unknown and open to speculation. It remains possible that intelligence scores are influenced by the non-neurological relationship we identified between genetically proximal bipolar disorder liability and genetic intelligence.

The implications of the study's findings are significant, considering that in previous research there is no general consensus on this topic. Furthermore, the potential to use bipolar patient populations as a natural experiment for bringing more insight into the presentation and protective factors associated with intelligence could inform clinical best practice. Specifically, this concept could help to make determinations for the cognitive ageing trajectories of clients themselves, but also their relatives and children. Further research recommendations include longitudinal investigations into the relationship between cognitive performance and bipolar disorder and related mood states. It is recommended that research continue to investigate the potential protective factors that drive intelligence and have diagnostics potential. Finally, future studies that seek to replicate these findings would be necessary.

What are the implications and what do the results mean? The study's findings demonstrate an interesting association between bipolar diagnoses and intelligence scores that are higher than the general population norms. By asking an important question about this widely disputed relationship between bipolar disorder and intelligence, the current study broadens the understanding of this relationship. This study's limitations, particularly the use of a medical sample, indicate a more casemix and less generalizable sample than in mental health studies. Given the impact of mood state on cognitive performance and an absence of test-retest reliability for intelligence test scores, this could also render the sample positively biased where hypomania and other high moods occur. Research based on population-level data, focusing more particularly on history of bipolar diagnoses, and separating by mood state may be a direction for future study. The finding is also accompanied by a pressing recommendation for further work using a prospective design to investigate factors that potentially drive intelligence such as neuro-protective factors or high early cognitive reserve.

9. Conclusion

The present hypothesis-driven investigation was initiated based on the hypothesis that both remitted and activated phases of BD could be associated with WD. Evidence from previous findings supported the association between the active phase of BD and WD. However, the direct association between WD and BD, in particular, seems to be substantial, and here attested even in the present investigation, although only on a trend level. Paradoxically, the association between WD and BD was not verified to be particularly high when BD is in the active phase, before treatment, as assessed in a number of studies reviewed in the introduction of the present paper. The fact that in a terminological and "psychopathology presentational" context could cover BD, although not the exact construct of BD with upcoming mood spikes, might offer a window to the understanding of the present and a new effect. So it seems that potential deficits in active phases of BD regarding social behavior and downstreamed functioning in a psychiatric and healthy population seemingly facilitate WD, unless the opposite direction assumes BD having WD as a consequence, leaving it unclear to which extent mere WD is a true antecedent of BD in any phase.

We did not find that among persons with BD, having above average IQ score was also associated with having WD, M, or ED. Existing findings suggested a decreased prevalence of BD in only some of the subgroups with a high IQ score. However, the existing findings must be viewed with caution, given that they were based on a limited amount of published papers.

9.1. Summary of Findings

There is no independent association between age of onset and WAIS-IV IQ. Greater number of depressive episodes is associated with marginally lower IQ scores in bivariate analysis, but this relationship is not significant and does not prove to be significant when controlling for confounds in multiple regression. In a pathway model, bipolar I disorder conferred risk for decreased IQ, but the severity and course of bipolar I disorder was not associated with decreased IQ after bipolar I disorder status was controlled for. In conclusion, this study found an independent association between bipolar I disorder status and IQ scores in a large, representative sample. We found no association between IQ score and the severity of the disorder or the course of illness. Our results suggest that the "bad patch" resulting from an affective episode as postulated by Van Gorp and colleagues is not supported.

In this investigation, the possibility that bipolar disorder severity and remission status could be associated with intelligence scores in a large sample of individuals was tested. Bipolar disorder is associated with a lower intelligence score on the Weschler Abbreviated Scale of Intelligence in individuals with bipolar I, as opposed to bipolar II disorder and those without bipolar disorder. The adjusted difference between people with bipolar I disorder and no bipolar disorder is 2.6 with a 95% confidence interval between 2.0 and 3.1 points, or half of a standard deviation in grab terms. Confidence in this result is increased by controlling for the possible confounding effects.

9.2. Limitations and Recommendations

Furthermore, as the intercorrelations between premorbid and current intelligence in BD have already been proposed, future research is warranted in order to elucidate the association between both healthy and clinically based sub-threshold phenotype variations to test hypothesis of "broad schizotypical" and "broad euphoric" phenotypes of intelligence. Typical psychotic features of BD include hallucinations and delusions in euphoric mania and reflect preliminary schizotypical findings that were also perceptually confounded by the subjects' primary psychotic disorder, a unique cross-categorical mixed state that occurred only during transient moments of years-long "broad euthymia.

Despite the support for the links between intelligence and BD, several limitations constrain the results. stated that participants included in intelligence studies were usually within the average intelligence range and with no mental deficits. This could have led to type I errors, making it difficult to observe differences in intelligence between BD and control groups. Consequently, in order to gain a comprehensive understanding regarding the relationship between intelligence and BD, further studies should be carried out including mildly mentally retarded and/or healthy individuals affected by BD—particularly unipolar depression. Moreover, as the present systematic review focused on adult individuals, the results should not be generalized to children and adolescents. Additionally, sex differences should be taken into consideration.

10. References

Felson, R. (2012). Routine activity and situational crime prevention. Criminology, 48.

Fedders, B., & Fedders, V. (2014). Table of Acentric Factors for Orthorhombic Space Groups. In V. Fedders. Smith Publishing Services. Official 22 Pages. Smith NAWSA.

Deary, I., Whalley, L., Starr, J., Whiteman, M., & Fox, H. (2004). The impact of childhood intelligence on later life: following up the Scottish mental surveys of 1932 and 1947. Journal of Personality and Social Psychology, 86(1).

DeFries, R. (1980). Genetic basis of reading disability: evidence from a twin study. Science, 210.

Cai, D., Khor, W., Ngo, K., Tansey, J., et al. (2016). CRL4 regulates cell size and TOFT complex lampbrush-chromosome assembly. Cell Reports, 16.

Bookheimer, S. (2002). Functional MRI of language: new approaches to understanding the cortical organization of semantic processing. Annual Review of Neuroscience, 25.

Bland O'Connor, J. (2006). Lifetimes of impact. A tribute to Dr. Karl Smith. Kansas English, 89(3/4).

Beedie, C. (2002). Representational distortions in self & other judgments. Unpublished Masters Thesis.

Baez-Llerenas, R. (2017, October 4). The interplay between bipolar disorder mania and creativity. Scientific American.

Aukes, M., Hienke, S., Cantor-Graae, E., van de Zweth, J., & Selten, J. (2012). Selfish brain and low self-reported inhibitory control: theoretical implications. Frontiers in Psychology, 3.

11. Appendices

4. A Residual Plot for the Linear Model The residual plot highlighted that there was no linear relationship between the variables of bipolar condition and the scores on the intelligence test (r = -0.02, p-value = 0.74).

3. The Demographics Questionnaire. The Demographics Questionnaire was used in the investigation.

2. Power Analysis Calculation Table Effect Duration 0.10 Small 0.30 Medium 0.50 Large Cost 75% 15 10 6 Benefit 100 hours 1070.47 hrs 642.28 hrs 428.19 hrs Benefit 2000 hours 21409.42 hrs 12845.65 hrs 8564.72 hrs

1. Institutional Review Board Cognitive Scale Hypotheses of the investigation proposed were: Null: There was no correlation between bipolar disorder and intelligence scores. Alternative: There was a significant correlation between bipolar disorder and intelligence scores.

Appendix A. Instruments

Appendices. The appendices contain the supplements to the essay proper and provide the readers with additional materials, such as instruments, details about procedures, methods, findings, and discussion builders related to the essay. In some cases, the contents may include comprehensive lists of a certain category, not included in the essay, but with the potential to support and inform related research.

The Relationship Between Bipolar Disorder and Intelligence: A Comprehensive Review of the Latest Research Findings

1. Introduction

About 1% to 3% of the population has bipolar disorder, according to modern diagnostics. Some evidence and theories link this disorder with the occurrence of creativity and genius. Two approaches to the assessment of intelligence have always accompanied each other: one that considers intelligence to be aspectual and another dimensional. This approach to intelligence is determinant for the assessment in three different psychological trends, i.e. differential psychology, genetics and psychiatry. Because of these three trends' increased interest and activities regarding intelligence, several studies on intelligence in bipolar disorder have been reported in recent years. Some research compared bipolar patients and control subjects, with other studies compared bipolar patients with different subtypes of this disorder. Intelligence assessment in these studies was predominantly based on results achieved at various intelligence tests included into global IQ assessment.

The relationship between bipolar disorder and intelligence has been viewed differently over time. Numerous studies have been conducted to show a correlation between the two, but the findings have been inconsistent. Nonetheless, these studies give us insight into the potential relationship of bipolar disorder and intelligence, which is particularly important in psychology. As we move further into research in mental health and psychology, knowledge of individual differences and vulnerabilities are essential in helping people in treatment and welfare. This essay will examine recent research on the relationship between bipolar and intelligence, and the differences in intelligence among the affected subtypes of bipolar disorder, in addition to discussing these factors' potential genetic connections.

1.1. Background and Significance

Signifying the importance of the relationship between mood disorder and mental health is primarily significant to mental health, a domain chiefly focused on assisting with improving quality of life. Secondarily, and in the modern era increasingly so, it is important for intelligence research. Impaired executive functioning and less severe impairments in global cognitive ability are evident in those who are euthymic. That is, in the absence of active mood disturbance and in a state in which the individual's mental state is considered more normal. Furthermore, there is evidence that suggests cognitive impairment can predispose one to developing bipolar disorder. There is, as one would expect from a current diagnostic manual that is based on descriptive psychopathology, some overlap in the clinical presentation and course of those with schizophrenia, with mood disorders and with just cognitive impairments. It has been hypothesized, given the many years of looking, that intelligence could be the mediating variable through which these diagnoses manifest differently.

Bipolar disorder is a severe and persistent mental health condition which is characterized by periods of mania and depression. We have known from early in psychiatry that those with the condition are of at least average intelligence. In the years since, there has been a considerable amount of research into what the relationship might be between bipolar disorder and intelligence. Many theories have been proposed, and many studies have been executed. There has been some suggestive evidence, and some interesting studies that hypothesize about the relationship, but in recent years, findings had not shown a strong case for a consistent pattern to emerge. But research is ongoing, and new studies influence our understanding, so in reviewing the current state-of-play in this research area we generate ideas that will inspire future research and acting on this research.

2. Understanding Bipolar Disorder

Bipolar II disorder (BPII) is often undiagnosed and has been shown to be associated with reduced functionality and disabilities and a high risk of recurrence in adulthood. According to the international classification system, temperament is flagged along the mood spectrum. It should be noted that low to high-speed cycle levels are predictive of early onset of BDDB or hypomania. In BPI-II, the current level of the cycle is clearly clearer than in reverse. There are also signs that emotional intelligence can slow when organ dysfunction of BD and BD occur. Symptom severity can affect the quality of our assessment and the overall results. BD is known for its neurodevelopmental history of early exposure to many disabilities. Despite the presence of some articles on BD, there are few articles available that discuss BD/BDHR intelligence.

Bipolar disorder is characterized by abnormal mood swings interspersed with periods of normal mood and affect. This type of disorder includes Bipolar Disorder (BD) Type 1 (BPI) characterized by a severe mood, and BD Type II (BDII) characterized by a milder form. BD is a disease that can be very severe, depending on the severity of the symptoms that occur. BPI-I [BDI] is described as a mixture of drought and melancholy, in which the patient "floats" and has great difficulty distinguishing between these two effects. Future solutions to analyze the mind with appropriate pharmacokinetic techniques are the subject of

a growing number of researchers around the world. This
could be analyzed.

2.1. Definition and Symptoms

The previously employed common classification system, DSM-IV, for bipolar disorder has generally described four types: bipolar I disorder (resulting in significant impairment but without psychosis or hospitalization), bipolar II disorder (resulting in significant impairment that does not involve psychosis or require hospitalization), bipolar disorder not otherwise specified (including those with subthreshold manic, hypomanic, or mixed states), and cyclothymic disorder (involving mood swings that are less severe than those of full bipolar disorder and that do not impair function). The most recent version, DSM-5, separates bipolar I disorder from a combined category including bipolar II disorder, cyclothymic disorder, bipolar disorder not otherwise specified, and substance/medication-induced bipolar disorder. While we acknowledge the unequivocal value of sub-typing within bipolar disorder, meta-analyses pertaining to intelligence generally forego this distinction. Thus, throughout this manuscript, the phrase "bipolar disorder" refers to all spectrums.

A common clinical definition of bipolar disorder describes these individuals as experiencing an abnormal mood of elevated energy, cognition, and emotion, and often mood congruent psychosis that occurs at least once a year and occasionally impairs significant aspects of the patient's life. Our discussion here employs broader operational definitions of bipolar disorder that are often used in research studies. In addition to full mania, other individuals with varying levels of the symptoms of mania or hypomania are included. We outline symptoms of mania and hypomania (which are almost identical to those for full mania but less severe) when discussing the association of bipolar disorder with cognition.

3. Intelligence and its Measurement

A number of cognitive abilities comprise the larger construct of intelligence. Fluid intelligence is involved in the ability to solve problems without using any prior knowledge. Crystallized intelligence is the basis by which individuals use the knowledge, skills, and experience that have been acquired through prior learning. This form of intelligence is used in situations where prior knowledge can be applied to solve problems and differs from problem-solving based solely on reasoning ability. A series of tests of mental abilities have emerged over time and are the primary tools used to identify intellectual functioning. Intelligence tests may measure global mental functioning, but they are also used to detect variable aspects of intellectual function, including verbal and performance abilities. Varieties of interventions and intelligence and memory training programs claim to raise and maximize the human intelligence level. However, due to the methodological limitations of many of these studies, the efficacy of this form of training remains unclear.

Human intelligence is a multifaceted concept, composed of a wide array of types of abilities. As one of the most studied areas of human behavior, intelligence has been developed into a number of models in the psychological literature. The g factor, developed by Spearman, is considered the core variable of intelligence that represents both general intelligence and general mental ability. A wide range of tests designed to measure intelligence have been developed.

3.1. Types of Intelligence

Influenced by the ideas of Howard Gardner, contemporary theories of intelligence note that intelligence does not necessarily present in the same way in everyone, or in a way that a single value score can encapsulate. To capture this complexity, theories propose numerous different cognitive abilities or multiple intelligences. Gardner advanced a Theory of Multiple Intelligences, which asserts that not all forms of cognitive ability are equally important, since what is significant truly depends on one's historical and cultural background—what is called "divergent thinking" necessitates further study. Given that research in intelligence and cognitive science, such as experiments or measurements, you prefer and favour are much more like the kind of intelligence that you choose and value.

Intelligence is likely to consist of multiple dimensions. Based on a theory proposed by Charles Spearman, a leading figure in the early history of intelligence research, it has been suggested that there exists one "g" factor of general cognitive ability that explains most of the variation in mental performance across different tasks. In his model, a lower-order group of factors, known as "s" factors, make some contribution to the specific performance in certain domain-specific tasks. While this theory was influential in the development of intelligence tests and interpretations of intelligence, many more models and variations have been proposed regarding the number and nature of the cognitive ability factors that make up general intelligence.

4. Historical Perspectives on the Bipolar-Intelligence Connection

Although some claimed that those characterized as hypomanic were not really very good at anything, physicians who believe in an underlying synergy between bipolarity and elevated intelligence began as early as 1924. In addition, one reason that some papers "debunk" the connection between bipolarity and all possible abilities is the emphasis on the "cyclothymic" rather than full-blown hypomania, hypomanic, or manic symptoms when the question of high ability is considered. Historically, a given physician's treatment choices when it comes to hypomanic or manic patients could have influenced the odds whether the physician would have made a serious follow-up to observe the hypomanic individual over the long term. Thus, what we thought we knew about all patients with these superior skills and personality likely clashed with actual differential diagnostic features relevant to either outcome: institutionalizations long-term or the type of outcomes that allow individuals to use their gifts more or less well for a significant period of time.

The first reported connection between mood disorders and intellectual superiority came from Caelius Aurelianus, a fourth century Greek physician. Later research findings also suggested within the last 200 years that there is a connection between "insanity" or mood disorders and some forms of creativity. In a literature review, physicians have been noted for their philosophical asides and remarks that the "intelligent were 'naturally' more melancholic" because their great mental power could not help but seek the meaning within meaning, the "ora subora." Physicians of that time certainly had a sense that the higher-up in intelligence or education patients were, the more apt they were to be hypomanic or slightly manic from the very beginning of the study. Even though many physicians began to notice the connections between hypomania, mania, intelligence, and certain skills, other papers would debunk these beliefs.

5. Current Research Studies on Bipolar Disorder and Intelligence

In this very recent study, data on intelligence are taken from the World Wide Web, which is a big data source, and also, the relationship between intelligence quotients and levels of depression and mania is examined in seven countries in terms of seasonal changes. In that study, contrary to the expected assumption, no significant positive or negative relationship was found between intelligence and the level of mania. Furthermore, in parallel with the evaluation of data through machine learning algorithms, a gradual decrease in the intelligence scores of those with higher levels of depression in some countries was observed. In a study that is older and belongs to 2011, it is stated that bipolar manic symptoms can affect intelligence tests and it is necessary to be careful in interpretation. These and similar studies suggest that the first, crucial point to be considered while conducting the studies investigating the relationship between intelligence and bipolar disorder is the mood state. When the method and study designs of the latest research findings are considered, it is possible to see that such points are heeded more clearly.

Big data and advanced neuroimaging methodologies are used, and more comprehensive information about the cognitive functions involved is being acquired, thus the way we look at the relationship between bipolar disorder and intelligence is also rapidly taking shape. Mental health and psychiatric diseases have long been discussed in the studies of intelligence and creativity. However, there are very few studies in the literature showing a relationship between intelligence and bipolar disorder. It is thought that the reason for this may be related to the lack of measurement of state variables (such as manic/hypomanic symptoms) and the small number of studies.

5.1. Methodologies and Study Designs

More detailed evidence of the methodologies and statistical methods used to identify hypo-/hyper-intelligence scores is provided in Table 1 for neuroimaging-specific research that examines the brains of patients with bipolar disorder and looks for possible associations between particular patterns of hypo-/hyper-functioning and lower/higher IQ. Of the 207 articles that were identified as part of the search process, 44 met the inclusive selection criteria. The chief reason for elimination from the review was the lack of true intelligence tests as part of the univariate analysis within the original research's findings. It is clear from the review carried out by Dickstein et al. that the only condition stipulated in relation to univariate analyses was that specific test measures of intelligence be employed.

Earlier investigations into the relationship between IQ and bipolar disorder have examined data from large clinical groups diagnosed with the condition and healthy controls, and have used a variety of standard psychometric measures. Holistic approaches of this type have been employed to successfully investigate possible discrepancies in cognitive function between groups. The present review chose to select only articles that utilised common and well-validated measures of intelligence such as the Wechsler scales, as a primary feature of any new review into this relationship should be to gain a clearer understanding by focusing on the role of intelligence as opposed to a more general ability factor. The degree to which IQ measures can truly provide information regarding intelligence is also a key issue. The extent to which intelligence is general or subsumed within specific domains is still a contentious issue within intelligence research.

6. Key Findings from Recent Studies

Alongside this research trend, there appear to be two prominent findings from studies tracking intelligence and bipolar disorder. In terms of cross-sectional studies, individuals with BD achieve lower IQ and WTAR scores compared to a healthy control group, though results vary depending on illness status and treatment. Longitudinal studies primarily suggest individuals with bipolar disorder display a stable IQ, though this may change following illness remission. Few studies have identified an association between cognitive decline and bipolar disorder, and it is not yet clear how this is related to intelligence. Additionally, recent research suggests that IQ may be protective against the development of bipolar disorder, though it remains unknown how this extends to risk for mania specifically. Finally, few studies have investigated the impact of sex on intelligence and bipolar disorder, though emerging evidence suggests that diagnosis of mania in adulthood may interact with female sex to significantly predict an increased risk for cognitive decline.

Researchers continue to employ a variety of methodologies to investigate the relationship between intelligence and bipolar disorder. A prominent trend that has emerged in recent years is the utilization of longitudinal designs in order to offer insight into the dynamic nature of these constructs. In particular, differences in trajectory of intelligence subdomains have been identified in some studies, though results are mixed. This appears to suggest that the relationship between intelligence and BD is more nuanced and complex than otherwise accounted for. However, no recent studies have extended this line of research beyond adolescence to investigate the trajectories of intelligence, cognition, and weekday psychopathology.

6.1. Cognitive Profiles of Individuals with Bipolar Disorder

Conversely, neuropsychological assessments were sometimes ancillary to other assessment shared via a larger toolbox approach. DSHB remained consistent across both groups, with higher levels of depression and mania being associated with worse all-domain performance. In contrast, our study flips the examination of the impact of course of illness and between-group investigations around and instead found that poorer cognitive performance, particularly poorer attention and executive function, was already present in the mid-to-late stage of untreated first onset of mania. These results need to be understood in the context of previous independent literature where the DSHB was associated with between group differences in pre-operative cognitive function in mood disorder for some studies and cohort with those receiving bilateral ECT outperforming their unilateral ECT counterparts in post-operative function in others.

6. Cognitive profiles of individuals with bipolar disorder 6.1. Cognitive profiles of individuals with bipolar disorder. Greater understanding of the cognitive patterns evident in individuals with bipolar disorder was facilitated by the focus of a number of studies included in this report. Particularly, a number of papers assessed 'task-based' measures of cognitive function utilizing domains commonly impaired in bipolar disorder, such as executive function. In order to determine the pattern and specificity of cognitive impairment in individuals across a spectrum of

mood disorder presentations, a small number of studies compared performance among people diagnosed with bipolar disorder against other psychiatric groups or healthy individuals on task-based domains such as executive function and self-referencing.

Key findings from recent studies.

7. Challenges and Limitations in Studying the Bipolar-Intelligence Relationship

Given these advances, why hasn't the nature of the relationship undergone a comprehensive review and reinterpretation from both a theoretical and methodological standpoint? The reluctance to incorporate the new into the old can be chalked up to an outmoded—and increasingly outdated—conception of bipolar disorder as inherited primarily in the classic unitary, all-or-none categorical fashion rather than as a continuous multi-factorial quantitative genetic liability. The binary model does not take into account the etiologic and phenomenologic complexities of bipolar disorder, nor the many cut-offs that jump out from the phenotypic landscape. At the same time, it fails to explain the strong association between bipolar disorder and psychosis, the male preponderance of bipolar disorder in childhood and adolescence, the frequent co-occurrence of ADHD and intellectual disability with juvenile-onset bipolar disorder and persists in seeking immutable evidence of bipolar cardinal features even in non-refugee samples of large PET scans, etc. An unyielding adherence to the discretion model even as it withers away under mounting evidence is a barrier as ominous as one to investigate it in the first place.

8. Implications for Clinical Practice and Future Research Directions

Implications for clinical practice and future research directions: The outcomes of the presented review show that there is a plethora of factors influencing the current state of knowledge in the field of the complex relationship between bipolar disorder and intelligence. Consequently, any direct clinical implications are currently hypothetical and will likely remain so for some time. While there is evidence at the level of the individual that cognitive functioning is related to mood and other clinical aspects of bipolar disorder, this is still on a background of substantial interpersonal variability in IQ scores, which also makes predictions uncertain. Notwithstanding these cautions, the review highlights a few observations that already seem reasonable to take into account when providing clinical services to those with bipolar disorders. Our review allows for the contention that, based on a comprehensive examination of the current literature, an individual diagnosed with bipolar disorder and with 'moderately severe' learning difficulties (in IQ terms) or below may raise a concern for diagnosticians and may deserve a full evaluation and active support.

Conclusions: A complex, multidirectional relationship between bipolar disorder and intelligence has been observed. Our results prompt several valuable implications for clinical practice and suggestions for potential future research directions. The research in this area is inherently difficult, predictions about identified directions highly speculative, and therefore, newcomers should approach any future work in this context with appropriate caution and awareness of limitations.

8.1. Screening and Assessment Recommendations

On the other hand, a comprehensive individual intelligence profile assessment might be particularly important considering specific cases such as extremely low-IQ status patients, particularly dysexecutive individuals, or phenotypes heading to a clinical stage with high-scoring on ADHD and BD symptoms. Conversely, progressive intelligence-elevational phenotypes can show better premorbid adjustment, particularly if premorbid to initial intelligence decrements are modeled. Ultimately, there is yet room to systematically investigate how a less rote-like approach to intelligence assessment may further inform clinical practice and contribute to mental health professionals predicting illness outcome or creating a comprehensive treatment. Thus, a hybrid approach is suggested. First, cyclothymic or depressive adults or impacted children and adolescents are screened for intelligence and school performance. If suspected, the full global intelligence assessment is indicated; if positive, the much more detailed individual intelligence profile is recommended.

Due to the growing body of research evidence, it is increasingly recommended to assess or at least screen for intelligence in individuals with BD. Considering that cognitive impairment affects nearly 40% of symptomatically recovered individuals with BD worldwide, the brief assessment of global measures such as full-scale IQ might already be part of a good clinical practice, regardless of the variability in findings for

different intelligence dimensions and symptom-course
subgroups.

9. Conclusion

We coined the term "creative adhocracy" to describe a somewhat reduced executive function caused by illness in these people but used intermingled with an albeit diminished cognitive flexibility to solve complex, real-life problems and to be resilient administrators (CEOs, managers, etc.) and entrepreneurs. Those items were applied in a battery test with 196 psychiatric patients classified as schizophrenic or affectively ill. The battery consists of a sociodemographic sheet, identification, and labeling of facial affect portion of Amygdala Battery, applied to 59 patients. Yes/No task portion was applied to 102 patients. Cognitivity Index and Diversity Index were obtained in all cases. The IOAs for Cognitivity Index are at the upper 90% with values of P = 0.001 for both cross-section of patients. IQ was obtained in six male normals and was very high without significant between-group differences, although as in the case of all hominid species, male intelligence exceeded female intelligence.

In conclusion, this book was written with the hope of contributing to the discussion about IQ, premorbid IQ, and intellectual functions in bipolar disorder, one of the most challenging psychiatric disorders. The findings are all convergent, although some areas need further exploration, including the mechanisms involved in creating these cognitive and intellectual changes. These changes are, in general, different in manic and depressive episodes, and most people with bipolar disorder have IQ above average;

some of these individuals qualify for intellectual giftedness. There is a broad range of problems in identifying children with a high IQ, and many such children are missed. However, parents and teachers should be alert to the common—and some uncommon—indicators of a very high IQ in children with bipolar disorder.

9.1. Summary of Key Findings

The genetic and shared environmental links show that genetic effects that increase the risks for schizophrenia and bipolar disorder also decrease intelligence. The cognitive deficits in individuals with bipolar disorder and schizophrenia are genetically independent, with little evidence of pleiotropy. One study failed to find an association between bipolar disorder and objective cognitive performance. There is little evidence for self-selection into or out of higher education. There are only small differences in the distribution of cognitive abilities among students who choose courses in the arts, healthcare, and social sciences compared to the general population, equivalent to about a 3-point difference in IQ. In some countries and among some student groups, very large negative associations between creativity and negative symptoms are reported, up to -0.42. Despite the robust intelligent disadvantage of schizophrenia, affected individuals are significantly overrepresented among very creative individuals. Concurrent depression reduced the IQ of a non-clinical sample by 20 points and that of a clinical sample by 30 points (possibly too large an estimate, given that they were expecting correlations of around -0.32 and -0.48, respectively). IQ can also be temporarily raised. Current depression made scores on a creativity test no different from those of healthy controls. In older adults, songwriting ability and creative ambition are independent of both reported mania and depression in a large (n=61,000) Finnish adult sample. A meta-analysis of studies on the relationship between the severity of mood disorders and intelligence found inconsistent results. A non-linear relationship was reported, such that moderate levels of symptom severity were associated with creative achievement, but more severe disorders were negatively associated with it. A lower proportion of more able children than less able children change their names through deed poll. Only four individuals with extreme cognitive dissociations have been reported. All had been affected by some type of mania or mania-related condition, such as delirium.

Summary of key findings: Bipolar disorder is positively associated with intelligence. This effect is moderate, with a potential advantage of 0.68 SD, meaning that individuals with bipolar disorder may have approximately a 5-point IQ advantage over the average person in the United States, which is equivalent to graduating from college. High cognitive ability may act as a premorbid characteristic that provides some protection against the development of the disorder. Depending on the timing of the first episode, the association with intelligence may be present but smaller, and could be due to other reasons (for example, an environmentally driven ceiling effect from functioning cannot be ruled out for some studies). However, there is also evidence suggesting that the association between IQ and bipolar disorder may be partly a result of the study design. Longitudinal and transdiagnostic studies indicate that the association between cognitive ability and bipolar disorder may be smaller than indicated in cross-sectional and high-risk studies that aim to predict the onset of the disorder. This may be because excluding individuals from easier-to-recruit studies and those who die before being assessed may inflate apparent differences between risk factors and non-risk factors.

9. Conclusion